Embracing Motherhood

How to Get Pregnant the Easy Way

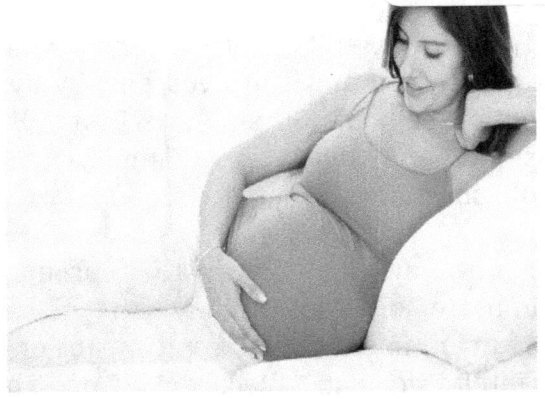

By:
Fhilcar Faunillan

Fhilcar Faunillan

the owned by the owners themselves, not affiliated with this document.

Table of Contents

INTRODUCTION

"A mother's love is forever strong, never changing for all time... and when her children need her most, a mother's love will shine."
~Anonymous

I want to thank you and congratulate you for downloading the book, *"Embracing Motherhood: **How to Get Pregnant the Easy Way"**.*

They say that there is no love greater than that of a mother's love for her child. At some point of most women's lives, we decide to fulfill that final endeavor of womanhood and that is to carry a child in our wombs, with or without a partner.

To reach that level of womanhood is something that is not to be taken lightly, as a mother you get to personally shape another person's life, another person's future. As a mother you get to love someone like you have never loved anyone before because that someone literally came from inside you, that someone is made of flesh from your flesh and of blood from your blood.

Because a child's first love would always be to his or her parents or guardians. It is up to the guardians, especially to the mother to maintain that love and trust and to make it grow. Motherhood is a great responsibility but it is guaranteed to be the greatest achievement of your life.

Multiple studies, poems, and stories will tell you how a mother can affect a child's life. It is true indeed that behind every great man is a woman and that woman is not that man's lover, instead it is always the man's mother. Jesus had his Mother Mary, even Hitler had a very close relationship with his mother given that his father was a drunk abuser, and Barack Obama, Jay-Z, Keanu Reeves, Al Pacino, and Shaquille O'Neal are just some of the influential, successful and powerful people on earth who were raised by single mothers.

And some of the most powerful women in the world are mothers, as well. Just to name a few, there is Hillary Clinton, Indra Nooyi, Pepsi's chairwoman, Jill Abramson, the executive editor of the New York Times, and Liliane Bettencourt, the owner of cosmetic giant L'Oreal. From this small group of people, we get a glimpse of how important and how powerful a woman can become by being a mother.

And although there are millions of women around the world giving birth to their miracles of life every day, it is undeniable that there is also a substantial number of women who have difficulty in conceiving their own miracle.

If you are one of those women who have fertility problems, then there is nothing to be ashamed of because you are not alone, it is a condition that is faced by thousands of women and it does not make you any less of a woman. If motherhood is your goal then there is no need for you to worry because there are so many solutions and options available for your convenience.

Also, be reassured that it *does* take time to get pregnant. It may not seem like it with the unbelievable rate of unwanted pregnancies, but really for most couples who are trying for a baby it can take from four months to a whole year before they can finally conceive. An average healthy couple has a 25% chance of conception in one month, so relax if you are not yet pregnant within the first couple of months of trying. Instead, take the time to prepare your mind and body, to enjoy your time alone with your partner while you still have it and to build up your nest egg for when the baby finally comes because you are definitely going to need it.

This is definitely the book for all those excited and impatient mother- and father-to-be's out there who need a helping hand in increasing their chances of having your own mini-me's sooner rather than later.

In this book, you will be shown a comprehensive how-to guide for a successful conception as well as the necessary information you are going to need to know to fully understand pregnancy and motherhood. There will be tips and tricks to enhance your efforts in the baby making process, there are also several do's and don'ts worth noting before and during pregnancy, applicable methods of changing your lifestyle to suit a baby-friendly environment, and the expectations.

If you are ready for this life-changing experience, then turn to the next page and let us get started.

Thanks again for downloading this book, I hope you enjoy it!

Chapter 1 - Beyond The Birds And The Bees

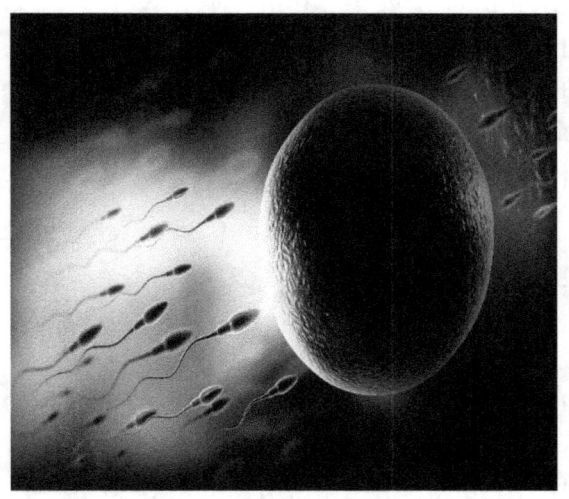

Knowledge is power and in this great endeavor you are about to take knowledge as key for a safe and effective conception and pregnancy. At some point in our lives, we have all been introduced to the process of baby making most likely during our teenage years where adults were in the hopes of scaring us into practicing safe sex. The operative phrase being "safe sex", but at this stage where you are more than just a hormonal teenager and ready to welcome a new member of your family, you will need to have a better understanding of a woman's fertility cycle or ovulation periods. Throughout this process you will learn that making love or sex is just a small part of conception and that sex is just a stepping stone, not exactly the entire road, to getting there.

At first it may feel like a paradigm shifting experience from avoiding a pregnancy, then suddenly wanting to try to have a baby, and then when you don't get the expected result of conceiving a baby despite several tries, you may start wondering how come nothing is happening. The answer lies on the woman's ovulation period.

Ovulation is that very short stage of the cycle when an egg cell drops down from a woman's ovaries to the fallopian tube to the uterus, where the uterine lining thickens, ready for implantation and for fertilization of the sperm. As said before, the egg has a very short life span that lasts for only 24 hours. What are the chances you are going to have sex during that exact day at that exact period of time? And just a fun fact especially for the males, ovulation is not the day when women are on PMS, that only happens after.

Ovulation occurs before the woman's menstruation or when the woman starts bleeding. Menstruation is basically the cry of frustrated uterus because the unfertilized egg is disposed of and the uterine lining that was supposed to hold that fertilized egg sloughs off to prepare for the next cycle, hence a *frustrated uterus*.

In a normal 28-day cycle, on average, ovulation should re-occur on the 14th or 15th day after the first day of your period.

15

But there are two major factors that affect the reliability to the 14-day period: first, hardly all women have 28-day cycles and most of the times it will vary every month and second, the occurrence of your period is dictated by the previous ovulation and it is not a predictor of the occurrence of the next ovulation. In one study, they found that even women with 28-day cycle varied on when they ovulated, only 10% out of almost 700 women ovulated within the 14 to 15 day timeframe.

Windows of opportunity

Now, you probably have a gist of how small the chances there are of actually getting pregnant. You may also start wondering how to conceive within that 24 hour window of opportunity to conceive. Well, no worries because experts have identified a woman's fertile phase.

The fertile phase are the days of your cycle where there is a slightly bigger chance of getting pregnant. It usually lasts for about two weeks or more. However, for women with irregular cycles this phase may be longer and not very specific. For a normal 28-day cycle, the fertile phase starts after the 6th or 7th day after your last ovulation – which means the day before the first day of bleeding from your period – until the 21st day of your cycle.

Even with the 16-day period, fertility experts say that you actually only have a six-day timeframe before ovulation where you have more than a 15% chance of getting pregnant. They call this week to be a woman's *fertile window*. And the best shot you got at a pregnancy would be the day *before* and during ovulation, but without special equipment or testing kit it would be particularly challenging to pinpoint exactly what time of the month that is, so let's stick with doing the act approximately a week before your predicted ovulation period. Sexual intercourse is highly encouraged during this time. A healthy sperm can live in the uterus for 3 to 5 days, that's why you have a window of one week instead of just one day thanks to the longer life span of the sperm.

Now that you have a basic understanding of how the fertility cycle works, the next chapter will guide you into utilizing these pieces of information to your advantage.

Chapter 2 - Counting The Days Through The Calendar Method

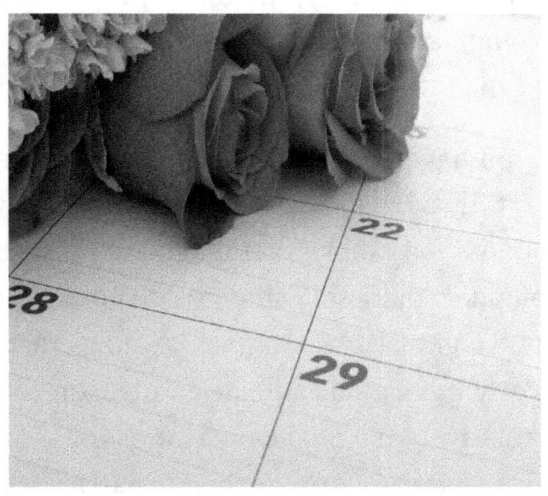

The whole process can be very confusing and is subject to a lot of errors in terms of noting the exact day and the exact number of days of your menstrual cycle. You actually have to spend at least two months monitoring your period to have a better certainty on how long your cycle is. No worries though because the goal of this book is to help get as close as possible to that miracle of life in your stomach. Hence, presenting the calendar method, a way for you to keep track of your ovulation and increase the chances of your sexual encounters to result in a pregnancy.

If you have browsed through the internet on this particular topic, you may have found that there actually are several calendar methods at your disposal, but you might also find most of them to be overly meticulous and strict. Also, there is a relatively big chance that most of those methods are erroneous, particularly because most of them are based on antiquated belief that a woman's cycle has a specific schedule it follows. It has already been pointed out by scientific studies that ovulation can occur at different intervals of a woman's cycle and contrary to popular belief: it does not follow a specific schedule, you can only have a close estimate to the pattern.

In some statistics, there is a 25% chance of the calendar method failing as a birth control. Hence, 1 in 4 women get pregnant due to mistakes in using the calendar method. This just goes to show that there can be a substantially wide room for error, but it also goes to show that 75% of couples successfully use the calendar method as well. So if you want to go the traditional and natural route of conception, the calendar method, with its 75% success rate, is just the right method to start you off.

Georgetown University's Institute for Reproductive Health came up with a *standard day method*, it was later modified by the American Pregnancy Association. A normal 28 to 32 day cycle was assumed when it was constructed. Basically, instead of scheduling the exact day of ovulation, these reproductive health professionals have divided the whole cycle into three phases:

1. The menstruation infertile phase: Day 1 to Day 6

This is the start of the cycle and it occurs during the first day of your period, so it can easily be identified and you can easily keep track. As discussed previously, during menstruation, your uterus is shedding the uterine lining that was supposed to shelter the egg cell once it was fertilized. So, it is safe to assume that no egg was fertilized at this stage and that no egg will be available for fertilization, hence there is less than a 1% chance of getting pregnant.

2. Fertile period: Day 7 to Day 20

A week after the first day of your period, the countdown to ovulation begins and the likelihood of your sexual intercourse resulting to a pregnancy significantly increases. Doctors recommend that couples engage in coitus during this timeframe at least four to seven times or every other day to maintain the health of the sperm.

3. **Infertile period:** Day 21 until the next period

For women who have regular cycles, the infertility phase typically starts on the 3rd week of the cycle. Obviously, this is the phase where ovulation is most likely to be over and the uterus is anticipating the growth of a fetus before shedding its lining, restarting the cycle all over again. However, for the women with irregular cycles the fertility phase may continue until this day.

Signs And Symptoms Of Ovulation

Now that you have a better estimate of when you will start ovulation, it would not hurt for you to have more clues to pinpoint exactly when you are ovulating, in fact being aware of the signs of ovulation would greatly increase your chances at a pregnancy. Also, if you are a forgettable person or if you have lost track of the number of days in your cycle being aware of your body is a reliable enough method to get back on the road towards conception. Lastly, this is especially important for women who have irregular or abnormally long cycles and cannot follow with the calendar method. Hence, in this section we will discuss some things that would clue you in when you are ovulating.

There are three basic bodily changes that you have to be aware of that specifically pinpoints symptoms of an ovulating woman. These are:

1. **Basal body temperature**: your basal body temperature is the lowest body temperature a body can have. If a woman is ovulating, the basal temperature usually drops and it increases by a 0.5 to 1 degree Fahrenheit two or three days after that. Hence, it is a precise predictor if you are ovulating or not. Moreover, it is very simple to do but it does require daily recordings to have a better grasp of your monthly fertility schedule. If you do this for a month or two, you can narrow down your fertility window until the day before your basal temperature heightens.

To take your basal body temperature, you have to use a digital thermometer or a basal thermometer – not a mercury one – because it is more accurate. You would also need a chart, you can make your own, just label the rows with the temperature numbers up to the first decimal place (e.g.

36°, 36.1°, 36.2° so on and so forth) and the dates would be at the top of the columns. Or you can download a template that's easily available on the internet.

To get the lowest body temperature, you have to take your temperature literally first thing in the morning. Before you even stand up from your sleep, reach for that thermometer and take your temperature. Engaging in any physical activity increases your body warmth resulting to unreliable data. Charting your basal body temperature would also aide your doctor in identifying any fertility problems you might have or if there is any.

2. **Cervical mucus:** Along with keeping track of your basal body temperature, your vaginal discharges are supplementary information that does not lie about the state of your cycle. Women

experience hormonal changes throughout the whole cycle and your cervical mucus is one of its manifestation. During the menstrual infertile phase, obviously you will have a bloody discharge for a few days. For the following days you will have a dry spell down there and then your discharge will turn into a murky or cloudy discharge meaning that your hormones are dictating that your eggs are not yet ready for fertilization. But when your cervical mucus becomes clearer and more slippery, almost having the same consistency of a raw egg white, this signifies that you are nearing ovulation because the slippery mucus is a way to make the passage towards the egg cell smoother and easier for the sperm to access. A woman is most fertile during or a day after there is no longer any slippery cervical mucus immediately after the previous stage. Hence, you are likely to conceive when you engage in sexual intercourse during the time you discharged clear and slippery cervical mucus.

How do you access your cervical mucus? It might be icky, but the only way to do it is to go directly to the source, which is your cervix inside your vagina. Some women have enough discharge that you can simply wipe it with a tissue and observe the consistency, but if not you have to insert your index or middle finger and take a swab to be able to examine it. It is once again best to do this first thing in the morning, at the privacy of your bathroom of course.

3. **Cervical position and firmness:** this is a bit more difficult to do and will take a lot of practice. With clean hands and trimmed nails, sit down along the edge of your toilet or bathtub and insert a finger inside your vagina until you feel sort of a barrier – that would be your cervix.

Before the fertile period, your cervix would feel firm and then as you get nearer ovulation it gets softer and moves upward, once it firms up again you have a 48 hour phase of ovulation. Once again, this would take a few months of practice before you can be sure if there are any significant differences in the firmness and positioning.

Both the male and female body are evolutionarily shaped for reproduction, at the core or at the most basic part of our humanity we are destined to reproduce, to make sure that our genes propagate for as long as possible. So, of course to ensure that we fulfill our obligations to our ancestors we have been equipped with sensors in our body optimized for reproduction. It may not be seen or detected both physically and empirically, but studies have shown that males subconsciously get attracted to ovulating women. It is because women release pheromones that attract the sensibilities of the male population.

On the other hand, because of these pheromones women have some physical enhancements. You may notice that your skin is glowing and healthier looking than usual, your lips become redder and plumper, your boobs become more tender and get slightly perkier, and many other things that will make you feel more beautiful and more confident to basically encourage you to look for a potential mate. Also, you would naturally feel an increased libido and become highly sensitive with your vision, smell, and taste this is to help you choose the best mate possible. Of course, these things usually go unnoticed but now that you know, hopefully this would help you know when the best time is.

Some Friendly Reminders

Using the calendar method and keeping track of your ovulation is one of the most reliable ways to get pregnant naturally and it makes you more aware of your body. However it does come with some warnings. Firstly, this is not an exact science and it would take a bit of patience for this method to be foolproof. Secondly, this method takes diligence and discipline to get accurate measures, be committed. Lastly, there is a tendency for some couples to lose their intimacy because love making may turn clinical and too scripted. So, it's important to keep in mind that it's not just about the destination, but also the journey. It can be frustrating not getting the results you want, but remember that you still have a partner that you love and care about, take this chance to keep that spark alive and

enjoy yourselves while you still have the
time.

Chapter 3 - The Fertility Diet And Lifestyle

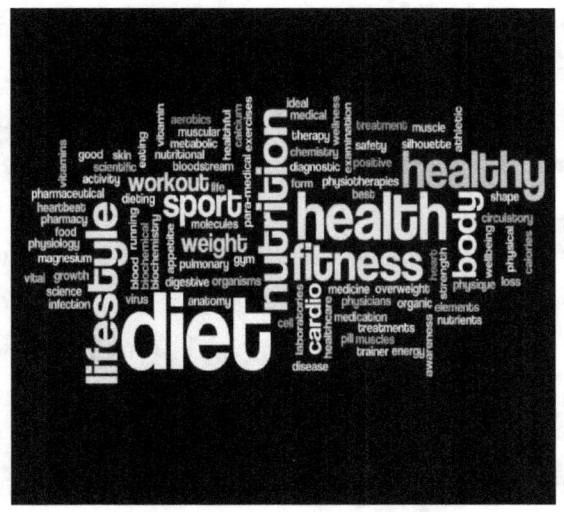

As much as you adhere to the calendar method and as much as you have a perfect 28-day regular cycle, if your body is not conducive for a baby you have a very small chance of conceiving successfully. Remember that your body is no longer your own temple, it is about to become a temporary home of a very small and vulnerable baby. Moreover, having a healthy body means healthier egg cells and sperms meaning better chances of getting a pregnancy and a healthy baby.

In this chapter, let us discover the dos and don'ts when it comes to your eating habits and lifestyle practices. Because if you want to conceive as soon as possible, then you have some catching up to do in making healthier choices. As you already know, this process takes a lot of commitment and eating and living healthy is one of those commitments that you have to take on fully. It's not like it would be too damaging for you anyway, yes it may cramp your style but just think of it as practice for when you have the baby in your midst. Would you want him or her to grow up strong and healthy? If yes then you need to set yourself as a role model towards making healthy choices. What you are going to read here should be applied to the two of you in the relationship, not just for the mom-to-be.

Well actually, a fertility diet is hardly a diet – in the popular connotation of the word – it is more about making healthier choices. Because unlike fad diets where less is usually more, a fertility diet requires MORE period. You need to build up your body so you are going to need a lot of carbohydrates, good fat, protein, fiber, vitamins, calcium and many other nutrients that will be specified in the following discussions.

Carbohydrates and fats may sound very unhealthy and for some forms of them they are indeed unhealthy and should, in fact, be avoided. But there is such a thing called complex carbohydrates which you can get from vegetables, whole grains, pasta, and brown rice. This food source is important because it provides energy to your body and your brain. Therefore you become more active and alert, which also helps in improving your libido and your mood. Good carbohydrates are also often accompanied with high fiber which facilitate the flushing out of the toxins from our body which in turn extends the life span of the egg cell and sperm.

Fats, on the other hand, is categorized into three kinds. The trans-fats or saturated fats and the essential fatty acids. Trans-fats can be found in a lot of processed food or any type of fat that has undergone unnatural processing while saturated fats are the oils that come from animals which is one of the primary causes of hypertension, heart attacks, etc. Both the trans and saturated fats are bad for you – whether conceiving or not, it is bad for your health. Meanwhile the essential fatty acids that comes from various sources such as fish, also known as Omega-3 fatty acid, and in nuts and seeds. The kind of fish that has enough Omega-3, like tuna and salmon, can be quiet pricey so you can replace them with FDA-approved fish oil supplements. You cannot just eat any fish and think that they Omega-3 because some of them may have ingested mercury from the water's pollution that they are even more harmful to your child, so just use the fish oil supplements. Also unsaturated fats can be found in slightly larger nuts like almonds.

The next necessary requirement is protein. Protein is the cell's building block, without protein we would not be shaped the way we are because it is necessary in creating genes and producing new cells. Not to mention giving us energy. Hence, protein can greatly help in producing more hormones to facilitate sexual intercourse and pleasure and also in the fertilization of the egg cell. Although there is a lot of protein from red meat, such as beef, red meat is also tied with several health complications that you do not want. So source your red meat from eggs, nuts, white meat, and seafood, especially from oily fishes and shells. If you cannot stand the thought of not eating any type of red meat then opt for the lean meat or lean cut where there isn't too much fat and oils.

Besides prepping your muscles with your diet, you also have to strengthen your bones with calcium. Milk is a great source of calcium, be careful though because consuming too much dairy products is usually discouraged for women. And experts recommend drinking whole milk instead of non-fat milk and any other types because the nutrients are still sealed in with whole milk, but they also recommend only drinking whole milk during your fertility phase not every day.

Now on to essential vitamins and nutrients to keep your health up on the scales. Vitamin C is especially important because it triggers ovulation as well as increase men's sperm count. It can easily be consumed in almost all kinds of fruits and vegetables, specifically in oranges, blueberries, mangoes, and carrots. Vitamin E makes for a healthier egg and sperm, hence increasing the chances of conception and survival of the fetus. You can have Vitamin E from leafy vegetables, whole grains, egg yolk, nuts, and oily fish among many other sources. We also have Vitamin B6, which is a common ingredient in prenatal vitamins. Like Vitamin E, B6 help your chances at pregnancy and avoid miscarriages because it facilitates the regulation and production of the hormones, estrogen and progesterone. The common sources of Vitamin B6 are eggs, bananas, beans, seeds, and salmon.

Onto some necessary minerals, a couple should have a healthy dose of zinc and omega-3 which have been linked with fertility issues by some scientific findings. You should at least have a 15mg intake of zinc every day, zinc deficiencies were found to be a common denominator in fertility problems. Zinc also helps in the production of semen and improving the viability of the sperm, not to mention that it will boost a man's testosterone for better and longer sexual drive. Fill up on your zinc requirements by eating lots of vegetables, beans, peas, onions, whole grains, and watermelon. Calcium can be found in milk, yoghurt, and cheeses.

Doctors also recommend that you start taking some prenatal vitamins even before getting pregnant, this is to ensure healthy fetal development and prevent any pregnancy complications. The first trimester is a high risk period and there is a big chance of having a miscarriage during this period and taking prenatal vitamins can help reduce those risks.

Folic acid is the first thing that always come to mind when it comes to prenatal nutrition that is because folic acid is proven to reduce neural birth defects in babies. Moreover, they reduce the risk for high blood pressure, cancer, and diabetes. The US Public Health Service recommends a daily 4 mg dose of folic acid which you can find naturally in fortified breads or cereals, whole grain breads, and dark leafy vegetables.

Other prenatal vitamins include **selenium** which also helps prevent miscarriages, and it can be found in carrots, tuna, broccoli, and mushrooms. Moreover, **magnesium** is necessary in keeping your womb and your baby inside healthy. It can be consumed from green vegetables, bananas, nuts and brown rice. Then, **manganese** prevents the development of any abnormalities and helps protect the fetus from harmful toxins, get a healthy dose by eating lots of fruits, especially strawberries, pineapples, and apples, along with some legumes, onions, and eggs.

The NO Go Foods

Keeping up with a healthy diet means that you have to sacrifice some of those junk food and sugar and many other food types that are most likely to damage your chances of having a baby. Here are the foods that you have to learn to give up for the betterment of your health.

Let us start with the big one which is caffeine. Yep, throw away that Starbucks cup and pour that coffee down the drain because caffeine is found to decrease fertility health by a whopping 27%. Moreover, caffeine impedes with your organ's ability to absorb calcium and iron which is essential to having a healthy pregnancy. And caffeine is not just found in coffee as sodas have high levels of caffeine as well; so yes you may as well put down that bottle or can of soda and never drink from it again.

Next, get rid of those refined sugars and simple carbohydrates. Candies, white flour, refined grains, milk chocolates, white pasta, and etc. contain a lot of sugar and carbs that are not good for you. These consume too much energy and instead of using the nutrients that you stored for conception, it will be used up to process all these bad food. Hard as it is to let go, you can have the alternative of using natural honey and eating sweet fruits instead of candy and you can also use whole grain products to fulfill your carbohydrate requirements. The same goes with trans-fat and saturated fats, studies found a significant link between fats and fertility where consuming these bad fats result in failed conceptions and irregular ovulation. Also, these fats will put your pregnancies at risk by increasing your blood pressure and blood sugar levels.

Processed foods basically contains all the bad ingredients including the refined sugars and trans-fats and many other chemical and artificial stuff we know nothing about. Processed foods like hotdogs, chips, cookies, etc. may contain hormones and chemicals that decreases your own hormonal health, it also contributes to obesity which is one of the common reasons why couples couldn't get pregnant. So, when you go to the grocery store make sure to pick mostly fresh ingredients and choose packaged products with less than five ingredients listed.

Soy products are also very damaging to human sperm, to the point of killing them or weakening them, because they contain a compound called genisten. Men should fervently avoid eating soy-based products like tofu, soy milk, and edamame. The jury is still out for soy and female fertility because they are a good source of protein and estrogen, so maybe avoid consuming these products on fertile days.

Lastly, limit your red meat consumption. Some people argue that red meat is high in iron and protein but they have also been linked with problems in conception. And experts recommend plant-based sources of these nutrients because they are more abundant there and they are healthier to consume.

Lifestyle Habits to Make and Break

If you are not yet a regular exercise person, then you better start being one now. Do not wait until you are pregnant to build up your stamina because it would be too late by then. Don't worry, you it is not necessary to go to the gym for a fitness workout you can just take up jogging or hiking or yoga as a hobby. In fact, high intensity workouts are discouraged, cardio is recommended and so is trying to strengthen your core. Once again, this is unlike the fad diets and routines. Your goal is to make your body more habitable or conducive for a baby, not to lose weight. Drastic weight changes only lessens your chance at a pregnancy, so seek to eat more healthily and incorporate some light exercises in your daily routine. Exercise can also reduce stress levels and increase the production of endorphins, your natural painkillers.

Speaking of stress, strain and stress have high negative impacts on conception and hormonal functioning. If you are stressed, your body becomes more focused in the production of other hormones that battle the stress and the reproductive system will be your body's last priority. Also, it strains the intimacy in relationships therefore reducing sexual intercourse. Another thing that could affect both your stress levels and your fertility health is your immediate environment. If you work or live in areas where you might be exposed to high levels of hazardous chemicals and too much pollution, then you will most likely have difficulty in conceiving a child.

Next, you might as well give up your vices now while you still have the time to adjust. Do not wait until you are pregnant or when the baby arrives to stop smoking or drinking. Moreover, these habits have very negative impacts to your health and reproduction. You have to make the choice now to either stop your bad habits or lose the chance at having a baby. It's all up to you to create a healthy environment for a child and smoking and drinking are not the types of habits a parent would want their child to pick up on.

And in setting up a healthy environment for a child, do make a savings account. Having a baby takes a sizeable chunk of cash and it's best to be prepared so while you still have the time, build up a nest egg for your child.

Lastly, make it a habit to spend time with your partner to improve your relationship. Do all the couple-y things that you have to do, relax together, and enjoy having each other in your lives because the best gift you can give to your child is a complete family.

Chapter 4 - Homeopathy To A Pregnancy

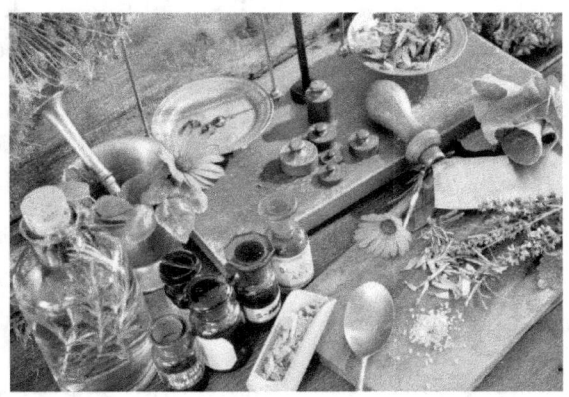

For the couples out there who want to speed things up there are available natural interventions that you could use as a secondary option. If the natural way of conceiving is taking too long or not really working for you, but at the same time you are not ready to go the medical route or take fertility enhancement pills then these traditional Chinese medicines might work for you.

For almost three centuries, traditional Chinese medicine still exists and most of them are, surprisingly, scientifically-based to cure or prevent almost any illness known to man. The ancient Chinese are remarkably advanced when it comes to medicine and they are even more remarkable because they use natural products and natural methods, unlike the commercial drugs we are so dependent on.

Their theories in medication may be disregarded by doctors due to the fact that Chinese methods are grounded on the principles of their religion, but upon further analysis people realize that their theories still make scientific sense and many have witnessed its effectivity.

You don't have to go to China to experience or apply these methods, but you should also be careful with counterfeiting herbal products and fake therapists who are not licensed to do any of the Chinese procedures. Fortunately, traditional Chinese medicine is already recognized in the field of medicine and is being regulated so there should be several clinics in your area that offers these kinds of services.

Acupuncture

We all know it to involve a bunch of long needles inserted strategically all over the body, it may sound painful and uncomfortable but rest assured that it is not. Acupuncture was used by ancient Chinese to stimulate "energy points" or specific nerves to retain balance physically, emotionally, and mentally. In fact, it is so effective that in a study in 2002 researchers found that women who receive 25 minute acupuncture treatments along with another fertility treatment were 50% more likely to get pregnant within THREE months than those who don't. The success rate is definitely tempting for you to give it a try.

Experts say that acupuncture allows your body to function more efficiently and allows the release of an egg cell for women who have problematic cycles. According to the wisdom of the ancient Chinese, we have a Qi (pronounced as *chee*) or a life energy that systematically flows throughout our body. When that energy flow is impeded, you lose the balance and thus become ill. Through acupuncture your balance and your life energy is restored so that you will experience a sense of well-being and your body regains its normal functioning, hence you women become fertile because your reproductive system is now in working order.

But in straightforward medical explanation, doctors say that acupuncture helps in the production of hormones that leads to conception. Secondly, it aides in the connection and cooperation between the hypothalamus – a part of the brain responsible for hormonal production in the form of neurons – and the pituitary glands – a part of the endocrine system responsible for releasing hormones to the blood stream – and the ovaries – where the is an increased amount of blood flow and hormones that stimulate the egg follicles. Basically, acupuncture is the oil to the rusty machinery that is your reproductive system. The ancient wisdom still applies in that it restores the connections (e.g. from the brain to the endocrines to the ovaries) for a smooth flow of energy (e.g. blood and hormones).

Because there are so many points in our body where the Qi flows, you can focus your acupuncture treatments towards restoring the reproductive system. The therapist can redirect the flow of energy from other parts of the body where you have an abundance of Qi. Doctors recommend going in for treatment at least twice a week for 30 minutes each. And after a few months you will have or feel the effects the treatment promises.

However, doctors warn that acupuncture would not be effective if you have any structural defects in your system or if you really lack the hormones due to age or other reasons. The Qi cannot flow where there is nothing there and make it work, so it is best to have yourself checked out first to prepare for any possible problems. And it is best to let your gynecologist recommend the acupuncturist or let him know who you have chosen so they can work together to create the best treatment plan for you.

Herbal Medicine

In the world of pharmaceuticals and chemical medicines there is an overabundance of libido and fertility enhancing treatments, but we can never be sure of their effectivity and the effects they can have to our body. Chemically and unnaturally produced medication are known to have side effects despite being effective and the biggest conundrum is that you never really know what goes in your body, especially since you are trying to conceive you might be exposing your future baby to harmful chemicals. Hence, the hype on herbal medication is rising because essentially the healing properties in the pills sold today come from plants anyways, so why not go directly to the source? Moreover, the herbs have a higher nutritional and medical content than the pills too.

So, to start you off to your herbal therapy here are some herbs that you can try that's found to be helpful in regulating the menstrual cycle, facilitates the production of hormones, improving egg and sperm health, boosting your libido, and help in dealing with fertility problems.

Estrogen production herbs

These herbs help detoxify your body of harmful chemicals that may cause loss or imbalance in hormone levels. Then they nourish the endocrine system to assist in the production of hormones.

- **Primrose oil:** is high in Omega fatty acids and helps in the synthesis of glands that control and regulate hormones. The oil should be cold-pressed from the seed of a primrose.

- **Sesame seed:** a very good source for essential Omega-3, healthy oils, and lignans that also promote estrogen balance.

- **Flax seed:** besides producing phytoestrogens – estrogens that detoxifies the chemically damaging xenoestrogens – this seed is also rich in fiber.

- **Red clover:** the blossoms of this herb is rich in vitamins and minerals. It helps purify your blood, detoxify your body from harmful chemicals, and is rich in phytoestrogens.

- **Dandelion roots:** this is healthy for your liver which is responsible for the removal of harmful chemicals in the body. It also stimulates digestion which will be necessary to keep up your strength when the baby arrives.

Fertility Cycle Regulator Herbs

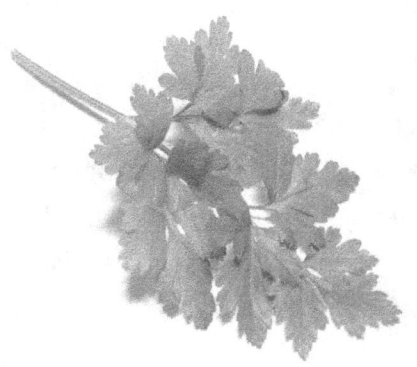

Having an irregular fertility cycle makes conception difficult because you can never keep track of when you will ovulate and sometimes you might not even ovulate at all. Here are the herbs that can help with this problem:

- **Dong Quai root:** this is rich in iron and it improves blood circulation in the uterus to improve the timing the menstrual cycle.

- **Parsley:** whether you use its roots, leaves, or seeds they are all a good source of Vitamin C which repairs any damaged tissues and protects them as well. And it is proven to bring on menstruation for those with irregular or missing cycles.

- **White peony:** this herb serves three functions: first it increases blood circulation to the reproductive organs, moves the blood around the pelvic area that stimulates uterine stagnant conditions such as absent periods, and it reduces the pain from cramping as it relaxes the muscles through improved blood circulation.

- **Black cohosh:** induces menstruation by aiding the uterus in its regular functioning of shedding the uterine lining, therefore easier for you to keep your cycles in check and your ovulation schedule.

- **Motherwort:** this herb is effective in reducing menstrual cramps and uterine spasms, other than being able to stimulate the uterus and improves its functioning.

Herbal Aphrodisiacs

The following herbs are useful in improving your sexual chemistry with your partner, not to mention increase your libido or stamina to increase your chances at a pregnancy:

- **Saffron:** this is an aromatic spice that was used by Ancient Egyptians to increase sex drive. What it does is increasing blood stimulation in the pelvic area and increase sexual feelings and desires.

- **Vitex:** from the berries of the Chaste tree, it is known to be the herbal female Viagra that enhances the overall functioning of the ladies' reproductive system, producing more cervical mucus, enhance sexual sensations, and increase energy levels.

- **Damiana:** by using their dried stems or leaves you can increase sexual pleasure and stimulate the circulation to your reproductive organs.

- **Muira Puama:** for men, this is the herbal equivalent of Viagra improving fertility and healthy erections.

- **Horny Goat Weed or Epimedium:** also for men for sustaining and firming erections.

For Health Egg Cells and Stress Reduction

Sometimes the cause of the problem is an unhealthy egg cell which prevents the full development of a fetus. This can be caused by several factors such as stress and inhabitable egg cell environment. So these herbs are designed for nerve relaxation and at the same time improved endocrine functioning.

- **Castor oil**: this relaxes, heals, cleanses, and stimulates organs and tissues of any of the body area. So focus rubbing the oil near or on your pelvic area and your temples to help relax stress muscles.

- **Ginger root**: ginger is known for its anti-inflammatory and healing capabilities. It also improves nutrient absorption capabilities and overall health.

- **Lemon balm**: this improves your body's coping mechanisms or responses to stress and is known to lessen anxiety and depression, both of which can be deprecating for couples who want to conceive.

- **Bee pollen/propolis**: this boosts both your immune and endocrine systems so that you will have better chances in making the egg cells catch.

- **Fo-ti root:** this is considered to be one of the most effective herbs when it comes to improving your overall well-being. This herb supports endocrine functioning and aids the immune system. This was also found to be effective for people who are said to be past the average age of conception.

Increase Sperm Count And Health

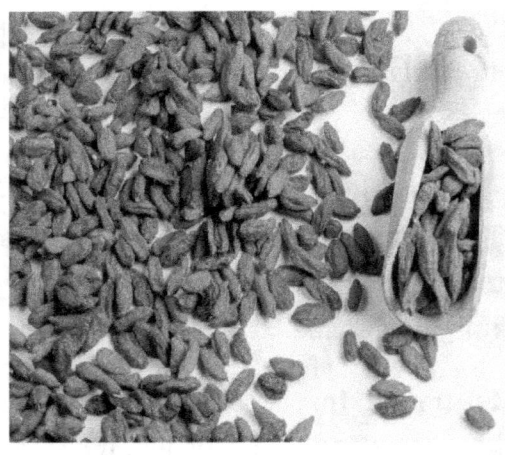

Because the egg cell has such a short life span, it is up to the sperm to wait and be prepared for its arrival to be able to conceive. On average, sperm can live for 3 to 5 days at best and the more sperm to compete towards the egg the bigger your chances are of having a baby. Hence, here is a short list of herbs that the male partner can consume to improve his sperm count and motility.

- **American Ginseng:** this is probably one of the more popular solutions to sperm count problems and for good reason because it is indeed very effective in not just improving sperm health but also sexual performance and potentially solves erectile dysfunctions. They also improve the functioning of the hormone-responsible areas of the body, specifically the pituitary glands, the hypothalamus, and the adrenal glands.

- **Goji berry:** this is important in the preservation of the sperm and in extending its life. They have properties that protects the sperm from hyperthermia and increase hormone levels to produce more healthy sperm. Its antioxidant properties supports liver functioning for improved hormonal balance.

- **Saw palmetto berries:** are natural solutions to impotence and testicular atrophy. Moreover, they improve prostate health and increase sex drive.

- **Gingko biloba leaves:** is very high in antioxidants and is also the most effective in solving erectile dysfunctions. They increase blood circulation to produce more hormones responsible for sexual drive.

- **Maca root:** increases libido in men resulting to a higher seminal volume and increased sperm count per ejaculation, as well as improving sperm motility.

These herbs are usually supplementary to improving reproductive health and as much as they are effective, but without the proper lifestyle habits and proper diet they will lose their effectivity. Also you can purchase these herbs in many traditional or herbal clinics around your area. Just make sure to conduct some preliminary research if they are licensed and FDA approved and make sure to consult with your gynecologist on the herbs you are planning to take.

Chapter 5 - Behind The Scenes Of Baby Making

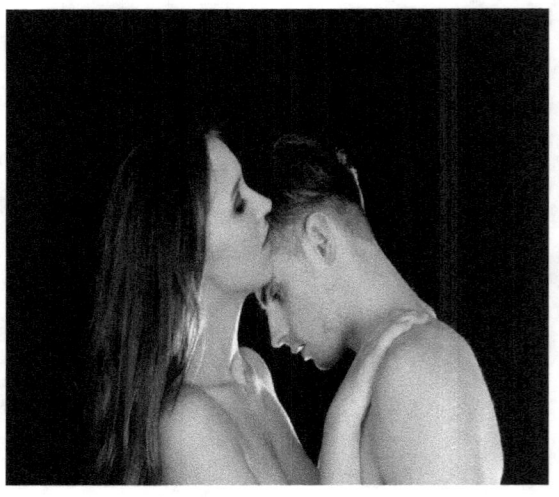

As a couple ready to have a child, you probably already have a lot of experience in the bedroom and perhaps you have experimented with several sexual positions in your time as a couple. Well, in this chapter you might be able to put those experiments to good use or if not, you will learn which sexual positions are optimal for conception. Also, here are a few ideas on how to improve your intimacy and strengthening your relationship that are definitely worth trying out.

Although experts say that sex positions do not actually have that much of an effect towards increasing your chances at conception, they can still have an effect on your sexual drive and performance. For example, the more men feel sexually excited, the longer the ejaculation thus a higher sperm count and higher chances for conception. Also, it would not hurt to spice up your sex life to improve your relationship as a couple, right?

These sex positions are usually with men on top or variations of the missionary position. It is to keep gravity on our side and lead the sperm in the right direction and keep it there. You can try or experiment with other positions that are not listed here, just keep in mind that it's best for the women to have elevation and deeper penetrations aid in producing orgasms which will make the woman's cervix spasm to pump the sperm towards the uterus where the egg is.

The Rock and Roller

Just from the name itself, it already sounds exciting. For this position, the man is above the woman in a kneeling position while the woman has her legs stretched above her head – she may place this on her partner's shoulders for more comfort. This is one of the best positions for conception because it allows for very deep penetration and it raises the pelvis of the woman.

Doggy style

You are already familiar with this position and it is probably one of men's favorite positions. What is great about this position is that other than the deeper penetration, doggy style is said to open up the cervix more than any other position. To make this position even more intimate, you can do the *Magic Mountain* position where the man hugs the woman to his chest while she is bent at the waist. Add some pillows for stabilization of her upper body, with this you can also stimulate the clitoris which increases the woman's sexual drive.

Spooning

This is another very intimate and romantic position, you basically spoon each other while the man is penetrating his partner from behind. You can try several variations of this as well for more stimulation and pleasure. The woman could raise one of her legs higher or clip it on her partner's behind. The intimacy of this position makes you closer to your partner that could improve your relationship.

The Butterfly

The name may sound delicate and sweet, but the execution is anything but this is one of the more adventurous positions you can have a lot of fun with as a couple. Using a table or any other flat surface that is high enough for a woman to lie down and be leveled with her partner's pelvis, have the woman lie down and raise her legs up to the shoulders of the man. The man will penetrate while standing up, holding his woman by the hips to raise it slightly. The raunchiness and excitement of this position is guaranteed to increase your libido and make your orgasms last longer.

The Plough

This is more acrobatic and will require stamina, especially from the woman. She will lie on her back, raise herself on her arms, and her legs are to be held above by her man. The man may stand or kneel behind her, whatever position is convenient, and hold her legs during penetration. The challenge will increase your blood circulation and hormonal rush which would definitely help in producing more pleasure and drive.

Where there are a lot of other good positions that you can try, there are also some that you might want to postpone doing. Purely on the basis of gravity that enables the sperm to travel faster to the egg cell, positions where the woman is on top or where she's standing up should be avoided during the fertile phase.

On the question of timing and frequency, men have the most sperm count in the morning after a good rest, so you can have a great start to your day by having morning sex. And you don't really need to follow a specific schedule of when to have sex, but it would be preferable to have regular sex, like every other day, especially during the fertile phase to keep the sperm healthy. The most important thing is to never make sex a chore, you should have sex because you want it and not because it is a means to an end. Take pleasure in what you are doing and who you are doing it with.

Also, remember to discontinue using your birth controls first. For the women, depending on the birth control you are using it can take from a few days to a few months before you become fertile again. Pills wears off very quickly so you won't have any complications with those, IUDs have to be removed by healthcare professionals before you become fertile again, but Depo-Provera or birth control shots take at least three months before it wears off so it will take you longer to become ready for ovulation. As a couple, you should avoid using lubricants and other oils because they may contain chemicals or spermicides that prevent conception.

Besides sex though, there are several other things that help couples increase their intimacy and commitment to each other. And because parenthood is such a big deal that it has the ability to alter the course of your life and the relationship you have with your partner, it is important to take some time off as a couple and reflect and prepare yourselves for what is about to come. With your acceptance and commitment, you will have no regrets and you will become better parents for it. Here are some ideas that you should try doing as a couple:

1. **Parenting talk:** it's not enough to say that you are ready to become a parent

because realistically nobody is ever prepared for it. Hence, it is important to discuss with your partner your expectations, priorities, fears, and how you plan to raise your children. Also, it would help for you to learn how to be good parents because good parenting does not come out of a vacuum, it is learned. You can talk with other parents and even your own to have a realistic perspective of how parenting actually works.

2. Extended honeymoon: if you can take some time off with your partner, go for an extended honeymoon. No, you don't have to go take a vacation somewhere else, but you can list down all the things you haven't experienced yet that you want to do before having a baby and just do it. When the baby arrives, you will have less time for yourself so take the time you have now to take those adventures and memories as a couple.

Also, this helps reduce stress and improve your sex drive so it will only speed up your conception.

3. Set an appointment with your doctor: if you don't have regular check-ups with your doctor, you should put it on your checklist even before you start trying to conceive. A pre-conception check-up will let you know if you have any health or fertility complications and you can be updated on the necessary vaccinations and vitamins. You will also be able to learn on what to expect when you are pregnant.

Be financially stable: it's not easy to have a child and it certainly is not cheap. As parents, you always want to try and give the best of everything to your child, but you can only do that if you can afford it. Not that being rich automatically makes you a good parent, but studies show that parents under financial stress are more likely to set bad examples to their children and use bad parenting styles. Without the stress and anxiety of financial dilemmas, parents can pay more attention on raising their children properly and can spend more time with them. That financial stability will go a long way in establishing a healthy relationship with your child and ensuring his or her future.

Chapter 6 - Infertility And Other Fertility Problems

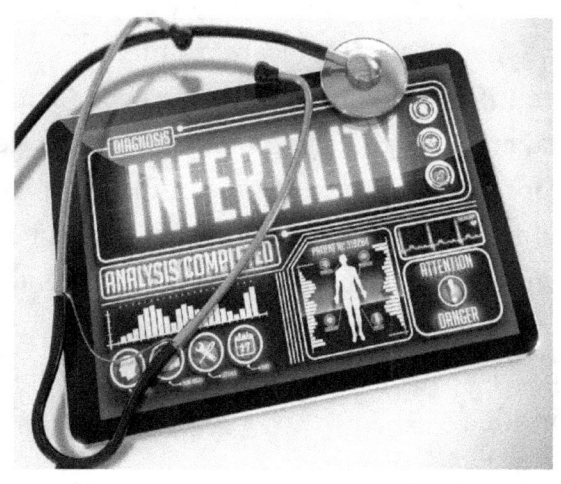

Disappointing as it may be infertility is a reality many women face around the world. No matter how difficult it is best to face this problem head on because the faster and the more you understand the problem, the faster you can look for possible solutions and alternatives.

Two of the most common indicator of infertility is a lack of conception and miscarriages. If you do not conceive, even after a year of having unprotected sex then you should consult with your gynecologist so that he or she can conduct the necessary medical examinations to identify what is preventing you from having a pregnancy. Having a miscarriage does not automatically mean that you are infertile, especially on the first try, but when it happens repeatedly it is already an indication of an internal problem. Here are the common causes and fertility problems:

Polycystic ovarian syndrome (PCOS)

In the US, 1 out of 40 women have PCOS. This is when a cyst forms in the ovaries rendering them useless until the cyst is removed. If have PCOS, you will have irregular menstrual cycles and there is a high probability that you will grow infertile. Other symptoms include excessive androgens which could manifest in severe acne, excessive facial hair, and male pattern baldness. Doctors have not yet been able to identify the causes for PCOS, thus they also have not found the exact cure for it. They do offer medication to help reduce the symptoms, such as regulate the menstrual cycle and ovulation.

Endometriosis

This is an occurrence where tissue grows outside the uterine walls and obstructs the ovaries and fallopian tubes which causes fertility problems. The tissue forms into cysts in the ovaries and could lead to ovarian cancer. Symptoms include pelvic pain, heavy menstrual periods, painful sexual intercourse, and painful urination and bowel movement especially during your periods. Pain medications are often given to patients with endometriosis and they can undergo hormonal therapy or conservative surgery to increase the chances of getting pregnant. Assisted reproductive technologies, such as in-vitro fertilization, could be used as a last resort for a pregnancy.

Uterine fibroids

Also known as myomas, uterine fibroids are non-cancerous growth along the uterus. Three out of four women have fibroids at some point in their lives, but they usually go undetected because they present little to no symptoms. They also vary in size and some come and go on their own. But for those who have symptoms, it often includes heavy and long menstrual periods, pelvic pain, frequent but painful urination, and constipation. Rarely do fibroids affect conception and pregnancy, but a certain kind called submucosal fibroids could cause infertility and miscarriages. So you will have to remove them first where you can choose to have a non-invasive procedure or the traditional surgical procedures.

Hormonal imbalance

Many women experience ovulation problems due to hormonal imbalance. This occurs when the hypothalamus of the brain or the adrenal glands of the endocrine system malfunctions or is disrupted. This causes you to have irregular periods and sometimes miss an ovulation which makes it more difficult to conceive. There are several hormonal therapies and medication that you could try according to the recommendations of your doctor.

Age

Women have the unfair disadvantage of having a limited number of eggs which they lose one at a time every cycle, so they have a biological clock ticking. The ideal age for women to get pregnant is in the early to mid-twenties, after that fertility declines and so is your chance of having a child. Past the age of 35, you have very low chances of conceiving and you are more likely to experience a difficult pregnancy. For men, even when they have an unlimited supply of sperm they also face problems with sperm motility, libido, and erectile dysfunctions.

CONCLUSION

"Being a mother is learning about strengths you didn't know you had, and dealing with fears you didn't know existed."
~ Linda Wooten

As a thank you for reading through this book, here is a checklist to start you off on your way to parenthood:

1. Visit your doctor for a preconception check-up and screening for possible complications.

2. Start eating healthy, balanced, and nutritious food.

3. Start an exercise routine.

4. Stop drinking alcohol, coffee, and sodas. Stop smoking. And don't do drugs.

5. Consume your daily requirements of prenatal vitamins and minerals.

6. Keep track of your fertility cycle.

7. Have enjoyable and pleasurable sex regularly.

8. Go on fun, spontaneous, and intimate adventures with your partner.

9. As much as possible, use natural supplements and methods such as acupuncture and herbal medicines.

10. Learn how to be a parent.

Hopefully this book is able to help you in your journey to becoming parents. Now that you understand how ovulation and fertility cycles work and you are equipped with enough knowledge, tips, and methods towards conception, you may already go and multiply!

I wish all of you to become the greatest parents in the world and to be blessed the most beautiful babies there ever will be.

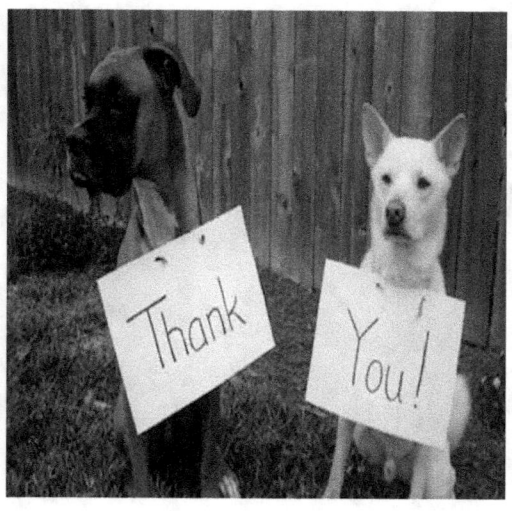

Finally, if you enjoyed this book, then I'd like to ask you for a favor, would you be kind enough to leave a review for this book on Amazon? It'd be greatly appreciated!

Thank you and good luck!